WHAT CAUSES ALLERGIES?

Rae Simons

The Kids' Guide to Disease & Wellness:
Why People Get Sick and How They Can Stay Well
WHAT CAUSES ALLERGIES?

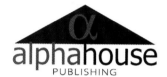

AlphaHouse Publishing
201 Harding Avenue
Vestal, NY 13850

First Printing

9 8 7 6 5 4 3 2 1

ISBN: 978-1-934970-18-8
ISBN (series): 978-1-934970-11-9
Library of Congress Control Number: 2008930676

Author: Simons, Rae

Cover design by MK Bassett-Harvey.
Interior and cover design by MK Bassett-Harvey and Wendy Arakawa.

Printed in India by International Print-O-Pac Limited

 An ISO 9001 Company

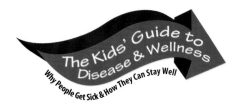

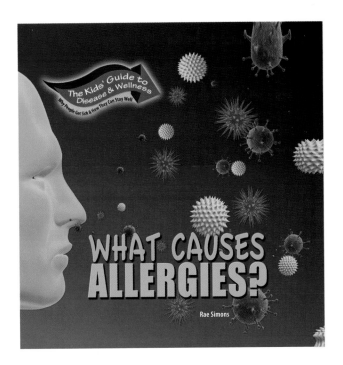

The Kids' Guide to Disease & Wellness
Why People Get Sick & How They Can Stay Well

WHAT CAUSES ALLERGIES?

Rae Simons

By Rae Simons

Series List

Introduction

According to a recent study reported in the Virginia Henderson International Nursing Library, kids worry about getting sick. They worry about AIDS and cancer, about allergies and the "super-germs" that resist medication. They know about these ills—but they don't always understand what causes them or how they can be prevented.

Unfortunately, most 9- to 11–year–olds, the study found, get their information about diseases like AIDS from friends and television; only 20 percent of the children interviewed based their understanding of illness on facts they had learned at school. Too often, kids believe urban legends, schoolyard folktales, and exaggerated movie plots. Oftentimes, misinformation like this only makes their worries worse. The January 2008 *Child Health News* reported that 55 percent of all children between 9 and 13 "worry almost all the time" about illness.

This series, **The Kids' Guide to Disease and Wellness**, offers readers clear information on various illnesses and conditions, as well as the immunizations that can prevent many diseases. The books dispel the myths with clearly presented facts and colorful, accurate illustrations. Better yet, these books will help kids understand not only illness—but also what they can do to stay as healthy as possible.

—*Dr. Elise Berlan*

Just The Facts

- Allergies are the result of your body's overactive immune system.

- Mucous membranes are your body's internal defense system. Allergies trigger these defense systems more often than is helpful.

- Your body has adrenal glands that help balance the histamines created by your allergic reaction.

- Some allergic reactions are triggered just by an allergen touching your skin.

- Some food allergies are life-threatening, but others are not so serious.

- A doctor who deals with allergies is called an allergist. An allergist can help you decide how best to treat your allergies—with a change in diet, medication, or maybe a natural solution.

What Is an Allergy?

You've probably heard people say, "I'm not sick. It's just an allergy." But the truth is, allergies can make people feel pretty sick.

Allergies are caused by your body's immune system malfunctioning. Your immune system is designed to attack harmful substances like bacteria and viruses. But with allergies, your body launches an assault on substances that are basically harmless, such as flower pollen, mold, dust, pet saliva and dander, certain foods, or medications.

8

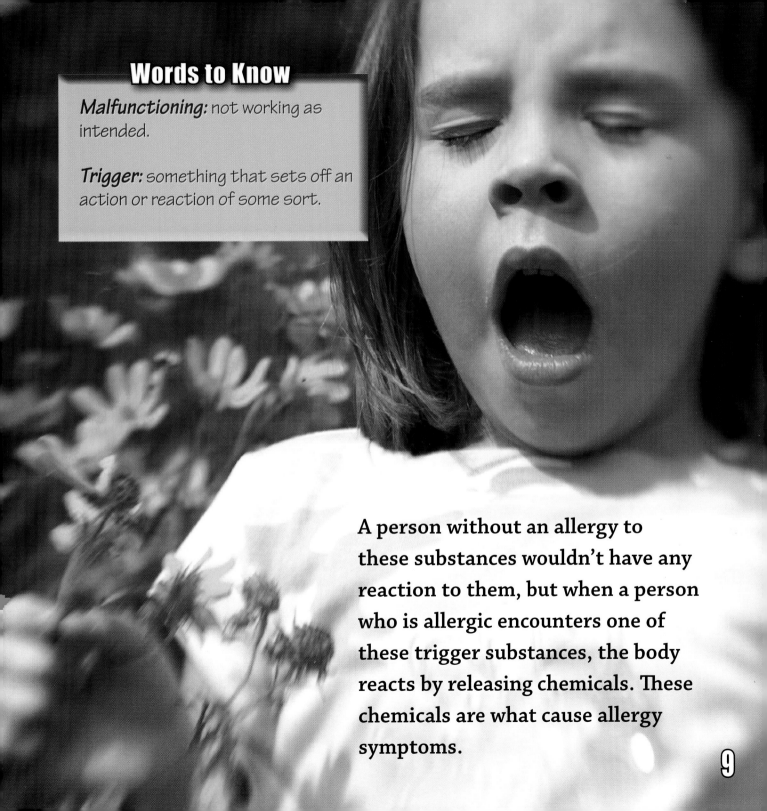

Words to Know

Malfunctioning: not working as intended.

Trigger: something that sets off an action or reaction of some sort.

A person without an allergy to these substances wouldn't have any reaction to them, but when a person who is allergic encounters one of these trigger substances, the body reacts by releasing chemicals. These chemicals are what cause allergy symptoms.

Your Body's Defense System

Your body is built to fight off invaders. When a germ or other foreign substance gets inside your body, your body's immune system launches a counterattack. The organs shown on the next page are all part of the immune system. Antibodies are the foot soldiers in your body's war against invaders.

Words to Know

Organs: body parts that serve a special function or functions (such as your heart or lungs)

Exposure: a condition where someone or something is laid open to or put in the presence of some influence.

Antibodies are designed to surround the invading cells, bind to them, and destroy them. When a person has an allergy, however, the antibodies bind to what would normally be a harmless substance. The antibodies then release chemicals. It's these chemicals that actually cause the symptoms—like sneezing or a rash—that we think of as an allergy.

The more times a person is exposed to an allergen, the more antibodies build up. That's why allergic reactions may not show up the first time a person is exposed to something—and why reactions tend to get worse with each exposure.

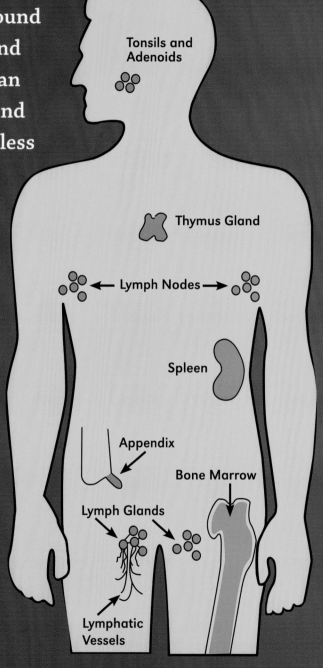

Tonsils and Adenoids

Thymus Gland

← Lymph Nodes →

Spleen

Appendix

Bone Marrow

Lymph Glands

Lymphatic Vessels

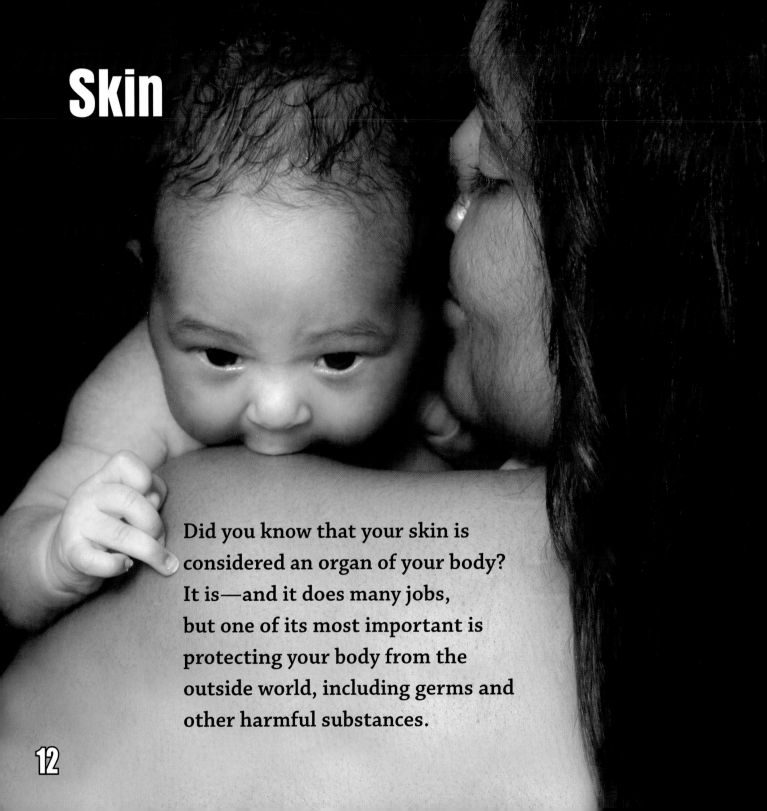

Skin

Did you know that your skin is considered an organ of your body? It is—and it does many jobs, but one of its most important is protecting your body from the outside world, including germs and other harmful substances.

Your skin is like the wall around the fort: it's what keeps the enemy soldiers from getting inside. But your skin is not just a solid wall. It also has tiny openings called pores. Sweat is released from these to help keep you cool—and if dirt or germs get inside the pores, your body's immune system steps up to do its job.

This means that if you're allergic to something you touch—like latex, the chemicals in soap or cosmetics, or certain metals—your body will send out antibodies, which in turn will release the chemicals that cause an allergic reaction—in this case, an itchy rash on your skin.

Sometimes rashes can also be caused by an allergic reaction to something you've eaten.

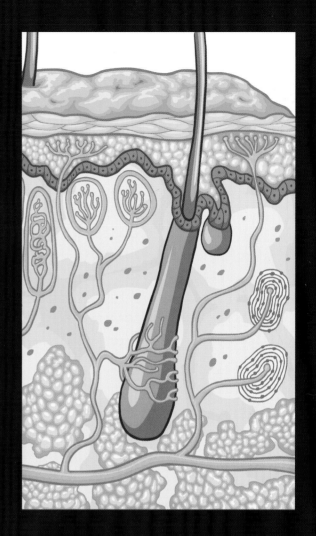

Words to Know

Latex: rubber, the thin material used to make surgical gloves. Latex is also sometimes used to stuff pillows and toys.

Mucous Membranes

Your skin protects your body on the outside—and on the inside, your mucous membranes do the same job. They're the thin linings of your nose, throat, esophagus (shown on the page to the right), and many other body organs. These membranes produce mucus, a thick, slippery fluid that keeps the membranes moist.

Your mucous membranes act a little like one of those sticky papers that catch flies. Germs, dust, and dirt stick to the mucus. This is another part of your body's defense system.

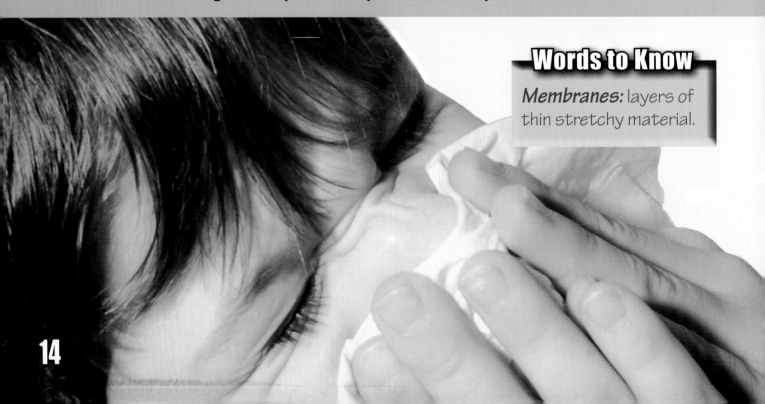

Words to Know

Membranes: layers of thin stretchy material.

If you have an allergy, however, to something like dust or pollen, when the allergen gets stuck to the mucous membranes, your body will react by triggering antibodies that in turn release those annoying chemicals. The end result will be this: your mucous membranes swell. They produce more mucus. Your nose feels stuffy. Your eyes get watery. Your nose will drip. Sometimes, especially with an allergen that you've eaten, the lining of your throat or lungs will swell.

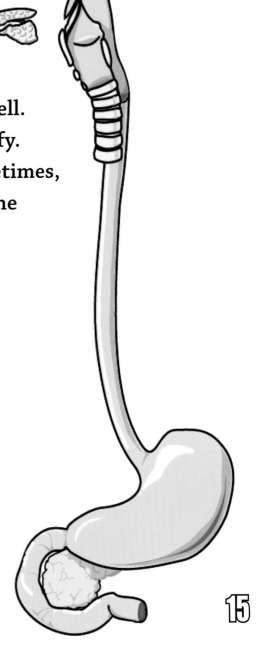

Did You Know?

Doctors recommend that people with hay fever (or other allergies to airborne allergens) wash their hair at night. This is because the pollen and dust can stick to your hair. Then when you sleep, it settles on your pillow, and you end up breathing it in all night. But if you wash it out of your hair before you go to sleep, the air you breathe will be cleaner.

Another tip: don't put fans in windows at night, sucking in air from outside, since this pulls in outdoor allergens such as pollen.

Lymphatic System

The lymphatic system (shown on the page to the right) consists of organs, ducts, and nodes. A clear, watery fluid called lymph flows through the lymphatic system, carrying white blood cells (the cells that launch immune responses) throughout the body. These immune cells are also called lymphocytes. They help make the antibodies that protect the body against invaders like viruses and bacteria.

Did You Know?

The lymphatic system is different from the blood system in that the blood continually circulates through each part of the body, pushed by a pump (your heart)—while lymph just drains from each part. Movement and exercise are needed to move along the contents of the lymph system. This another reason exercise is good for you—it can make your lymphatic system function better.

Words to Know

Ducts: small openings through which a fluid flows from one place into another.

Nodes: oval masses of lymph cells that act as filters.

16

When you have an infection, your lymph nodes often swell and become painful. This is because they're working overtime to fight off germs. Swollen lymph notes are actually a sign that your body is doing its job.

When you have an allergy, though, your lymph nodes may also become swollen in reaction to the allergen.

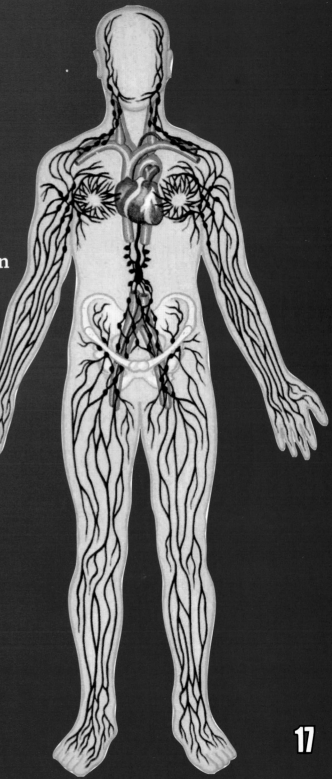

White Blood Cells

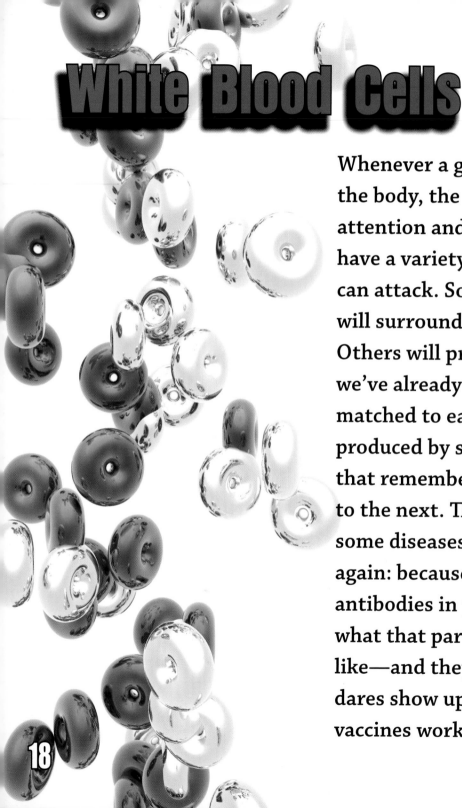

Whenever a germ or infection enters the body, the white blood cells snap to attention and race to do battle. They have a variety of ways by which they can attack. Some white blood cells will will surround and eat the bacteria. Others will produce the antibodies we've already talked about, which are matched to each enemy. These are produced by special "memory cells" that remember enemies from one time to the next. This is why once you've had some diseases, you can't catch them again: because you already have antibodies in place that "remember" what that particular enemy looks like—and they're ready to kill it if it dares show up again. This is also how vaccines work.

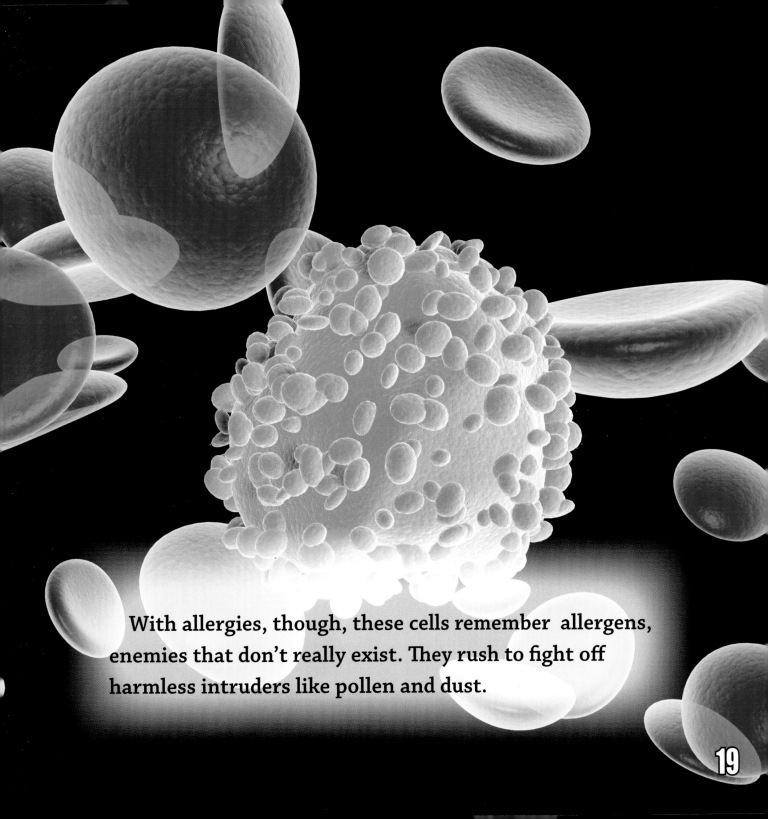

With allergies, though, these cells remember allergens, enemies that don't really exist. They rush to fight off harmless intruders like pollen and dust.

Histamines

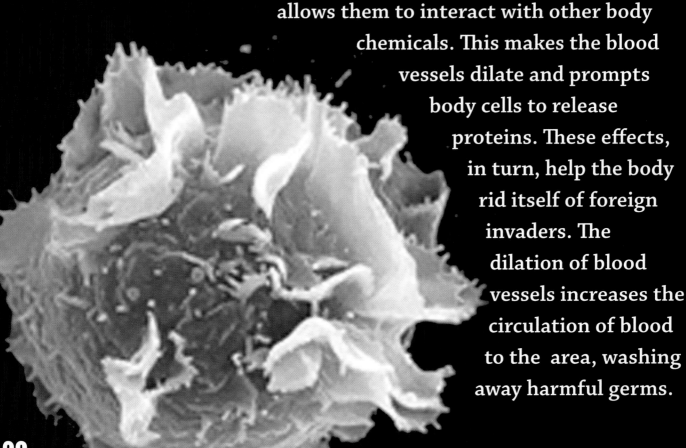

The chemicals that your immune system releases as it attacks invaders are called histamines (shown on this page magnified thousands of times). Histamines have a chemical structure that looks like the molecules on the page to the left. Their structure allows them to interact with other body chemicals. This makes the blood vessels dilate and prompts body cells to release proteins. These effects, in turn, help the body rid itself of foreign invaders. The dilation of blood vessels increases the circulation of blood to the area, washing away harmful germs.

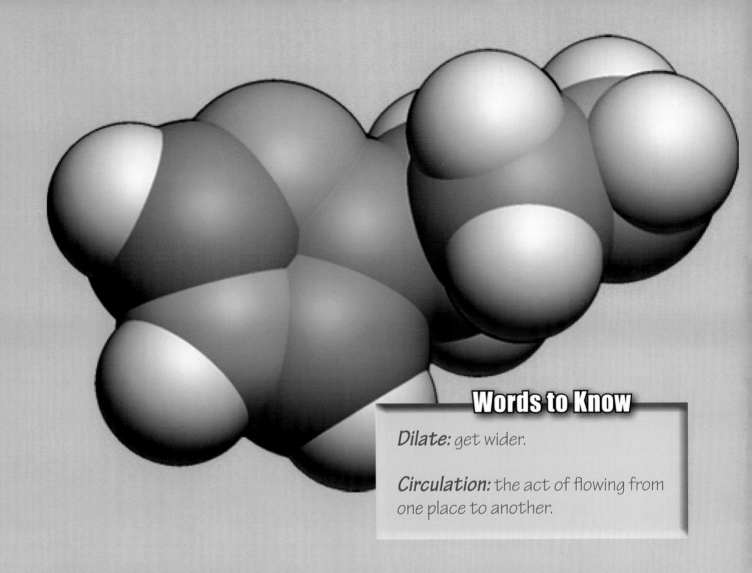

Words to Know

Dilate: get wider.

Circulation: the act of flowing from one place to another.

The release of proteins from cells brings even more white blood cells to the area. In response to all this, the "battleground" becomes red and swollen. This is all normal and helpful when your body is fighting off a germ of some sort—but it's not so helpful when you have an allergy and the same reactions occur!

Adrenal Glands

Your adrenal glands are located directly above each kidney (shown to the right). They help your body regulate its stress response. One way they do this is by making a chemical called cortisol. Cortisol is a hormone that helps control your body's reaction to histamines (the chemical released by antibodies fighting both germs and allergens). Cortisol is an anti-inflammatory, a substance that reduces inflammation. The amount of cortisol circulating through your body helps keep in balance your body's responses to germs.

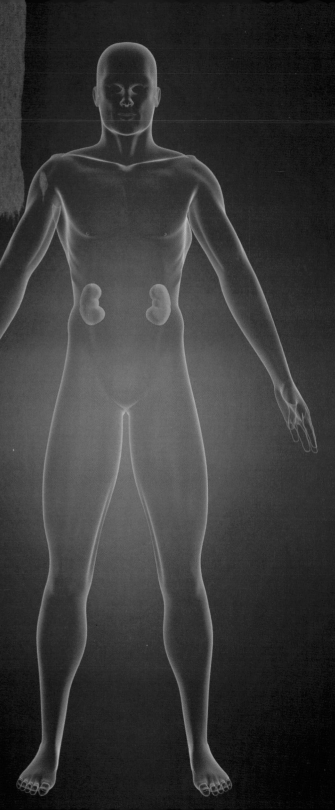

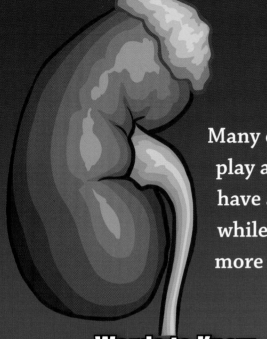

Many doctors believe that the adrenal glands play an important role in allergies. If you have allergies, histamines are released all the while you are exposed to the allergen. The more histamine that is released, the more cortisol it takes to control the inflammatory response. So if the adrenal glands produced more cortisol, allergy symptoms would be reduced. This means that doctors may be able to treat allergies by helping the adrenal gland produce more cortisol.

Words to Know

Stress response: what your body does to handle increased mental, physical, and emotional pressure.

Circulating: flowing, moving.

Hormone: a chemical your body produces that tells other body parts what to do.

Inflammation: when body tissues become red, hot, and swollen.

Body Temperature

We usually think that having a fever means you're sick. Actually, though, having a fever usually means your body is doing its job to fight off germs. Since many germs can't survive at higher temperatures, a fever makes it easier for your body to kill the germs.

Allergies don't usually cause high body temperatures, but sometimes they may cause low-grade fevers. A serious allergic reaction can trigger higher temperatures. If that happens, you probably need to see a doctor.

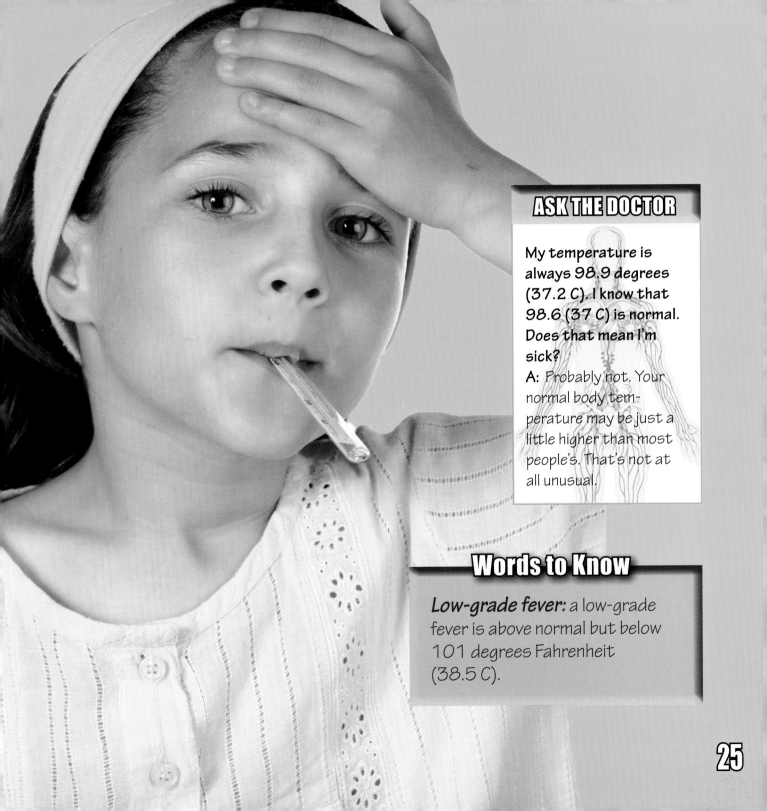

My temperature is always 98.9 degrees (37.2 C). I know that 98.6 (37 C) is normal. Does that mean I'm sick?

A: Probably not. Your normal body temperature may be just a little higher than most people's. That's not at all unusual.

Words to Know

Low-grade fever: a low-grade fever is above normal but below 101 degrees Fahrenheit (38.5 C).

Airborne Allergens

Many people react to allergens that come to them through the air, things like dust, pollen, mold, and animal dander. When people breathe these tiny particles into their nose and mouth, they stick to the mucous membranes and trigger an allergic reaction.

Words to Know

Dander: small scales from an animal's skin, fur, or feathers.

Symptoms that indicate you may have an allergy to something that is airborne include:

- sneezing
- a runny nose
- itchy eyes
- watery eyes
- itchy nose or throat
- coughing

Some people with airborne allergies develop asthma. The symptoms of asthma include coughing, wheezing, and shortness of breath because the airways in the lungs have become narrow from too much mucus and inflammation. People with asthma need to be treated by a doctor.

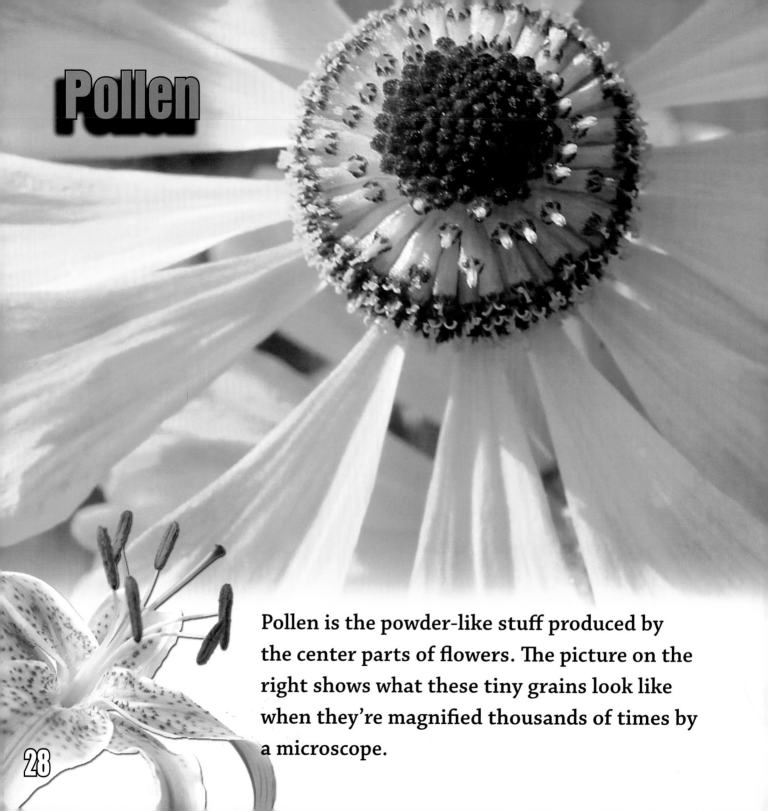

Pollen

Pollen is the powder-like stuff produced by the center parts of flowers. The picture on the right shows what these tiny grains look like when they're magnified thousands of times by a microscope.

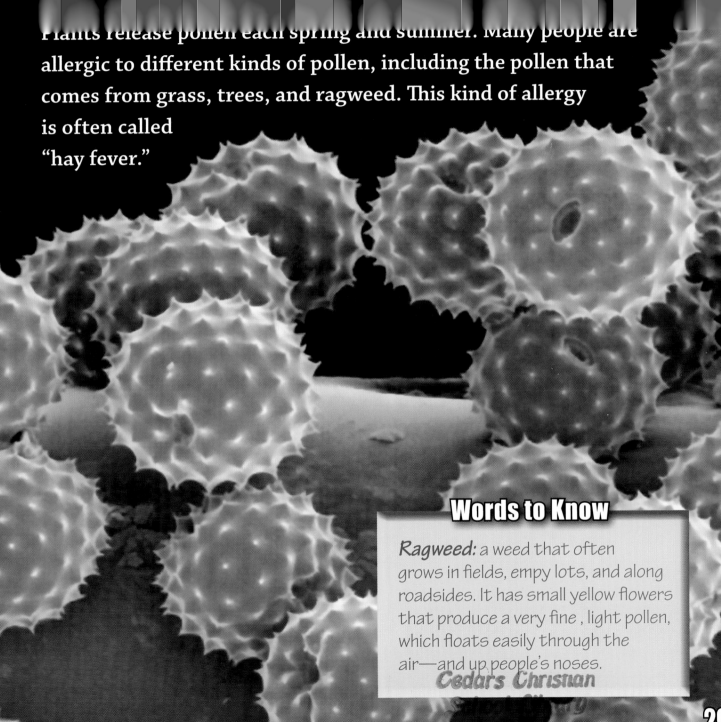

Plants release pollen each spring and summer. Many people are allergic to different kinds of pollen, including the pollen that comes from grass, trees, and ragweed. This kind of allergy is often called "hay fever."

Words to Know

Ragweed: a weed that often grows in fields, empy lots, and along roadsides. It has small yellow flowers that produce a very fine , light pollen, which floats easily through the air—and up people's noses.

29

Mold

Mold is that gray and black stuff that grows on damp surfaces. It's a fungus that releases tiny spores (shown in the illustration to the right).

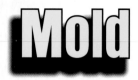

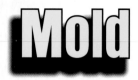

Words to Know

Spores: very small, single cells that fungi, algae, bacteria, and some nonflowering plants use to reproduce (instead of seeds).

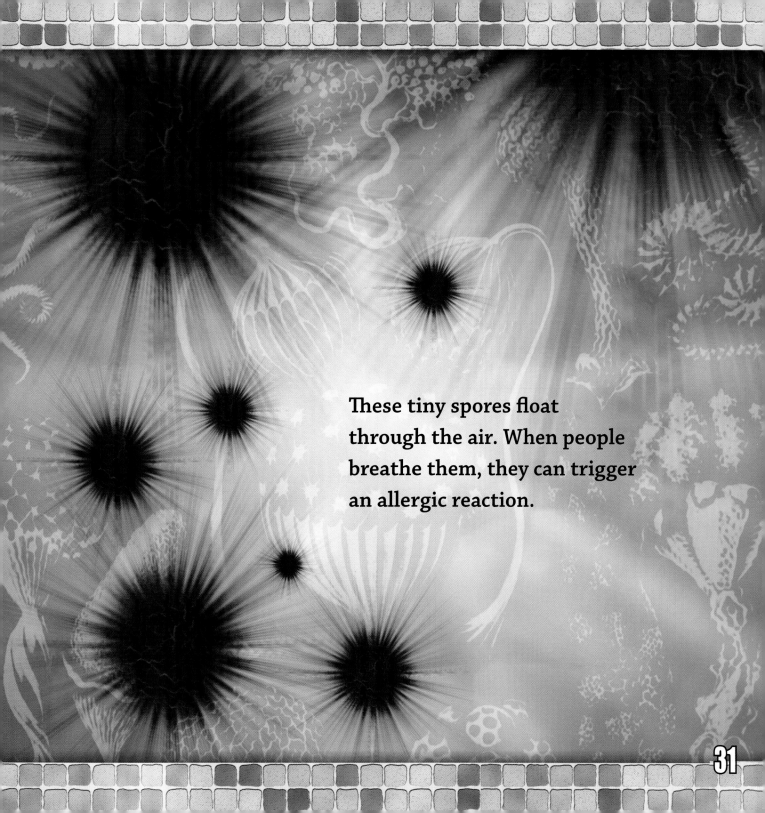

These tiny spores float through the air. When people breathe them, they can trigger an allergic reaction.

Animal Dander

The flakes shown on this page are animal dander, magnified thousands of times by a very strong microscope. Dander is actually tiny pieces of animal skin, a little like human dandruff (only even smaller.)

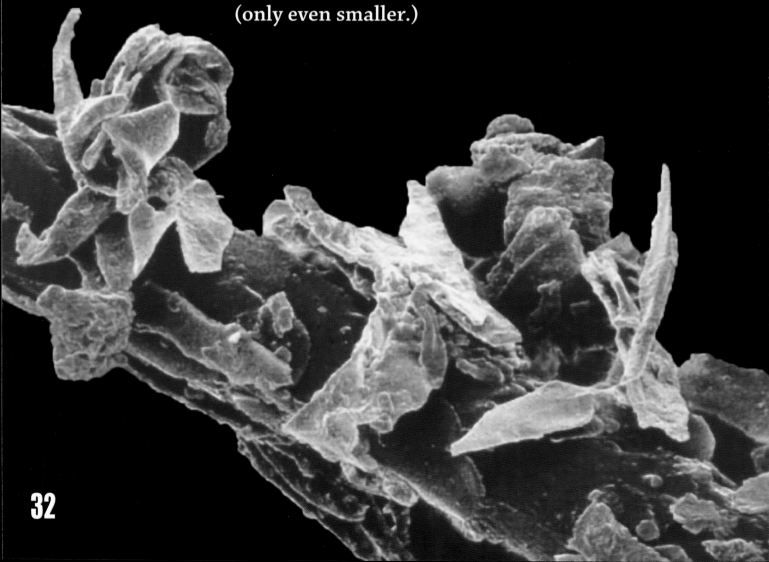

Did You Know?

There's no such thing as a nonallergenic breed of dog. All dogs produce dander. However, some kinds of dogs produce MORE dander than others. Dogs who are prone to skin infections have more dry skin—which ends up floating through the air and triggering allergies.

If you're allergic to your best friend, here's some things you can do: Wash bedding often. Mop hard floors and vacuum carpets every day. Don't sleep with your dog (no matter how much you love him).

Dander floats through the air. It sticks to furniture and bedding. And it goes up your nose when you breathe. If you're allergic to animal dander, breathing it triggers an allergic reaction: runny nose, itchy eyes, a stuffy head.

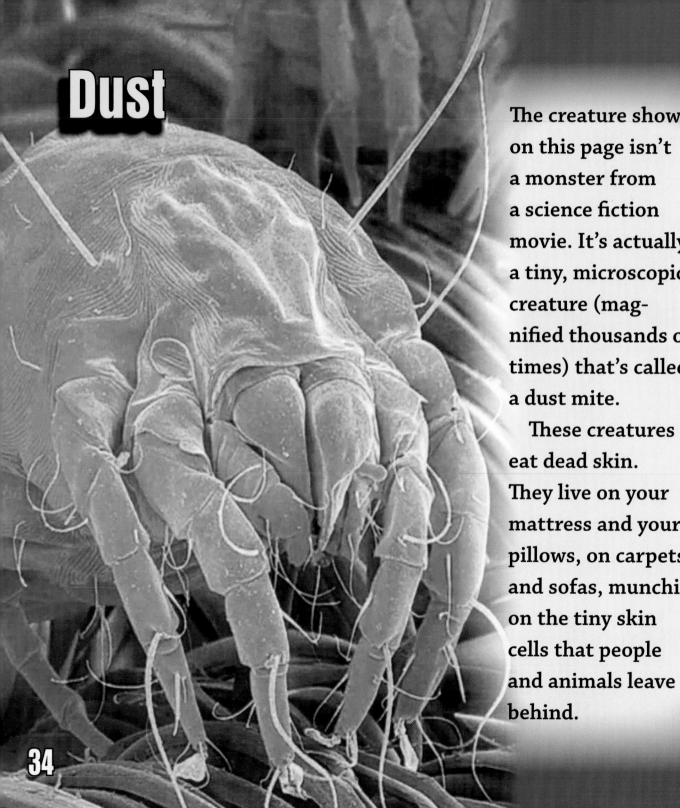

Dust

The creature shown on this page isn't a monster from a science fiction movie. It's actually a tiny, microscopic creature (magnified thousands of times) that's called a dust mite.

These creatures eat dead skin. They live on your mattress and your pillows, on carpets and sofas, munching on the tiny skin cells that people and animals leave behind.

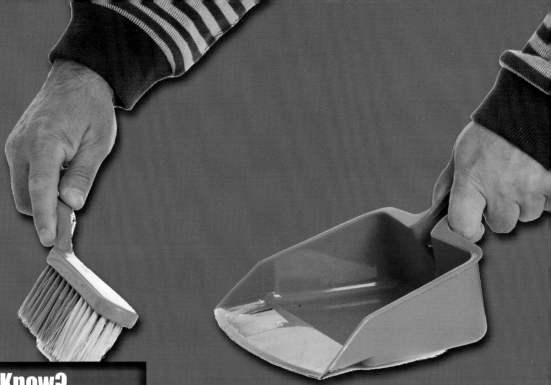

A typical used mattress may have anywhere from 100,000 to 10 million mites inside. One-tenth of the weight of a two-year-old pillow can be dead mites and their droppings!

Mites prefer warm, moist surroundings like the inside of a mattress when someone is on it.

About 80 percent of the material seen floating in a sunbeam is actually skin flakes.

As disgusting as it may seem to know that tiny bugs are constantly on you and around you, dust mites are actually harmless. However, their feces (poop) can trigger an allergic reaction in some people. Mite poop is so small that it floats in the air—and people breath it.

Chemicals

Chemicals are everywhere. They're in cleaning products, in perfume and other cosmetics, and in building materials. People with allergies can be exposed to airborne chemicals (such as paint fumes and cigarette smoke). They can come in contact with chemicals in jewelry that touches their skin. They may swallow chemicals on fruit or vegetables and in medicines.

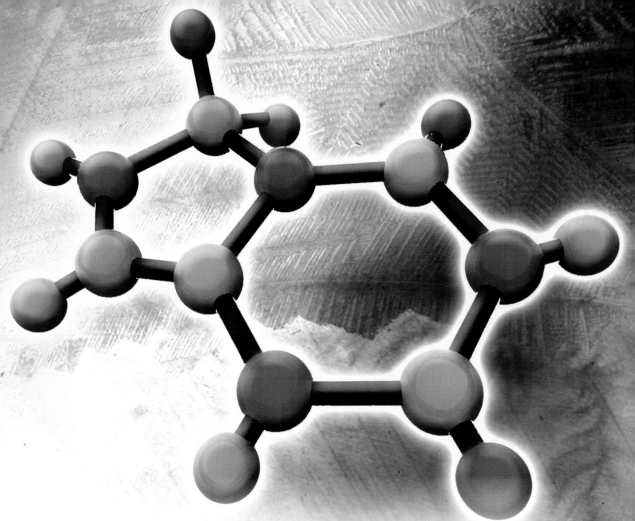

Some of the most common chemical allergens include: nickel (found in jewelry), some kinds of antibiotics (medicines used to fight infections), fragrances (used in perfume, lotions, and some household products), latex (rubber), blue-black dye (used in magazines, fabrics, and hair dye), and certain preservatives (used in eye shadows and contact lens solutions).

Contact Allergies

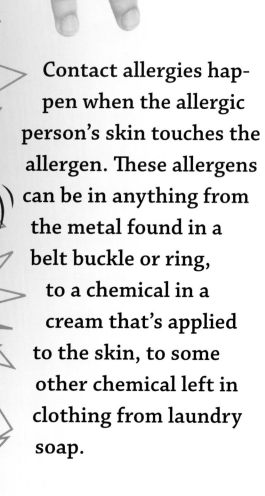

Contact allergies happen when the allergic person's skin touches the allergen. These allergens can be in anything from the metal found in a belt buckle or ring, to a chemical in a cream that's applied to the skin, to some other chemical left in clothing from laundry soap.

Contact allergies can be very annoying. The histamines in your body make your skin become inflamed and red—and the inflammation makes you itch. Sometimes the rash is only mildly irritating, but some skin reactions can be serious, with open wounds.

And scratching just makes it worse!

Words to Know

Contact: touch.

Plants and Insects

Poison ivy and poison oak are two of the most common contact allergens. Both plants cause a serious weepy rash. Almost everyone in the world is allergic to these plants (though usually you don't react the first time you come in contact with them). So when you see 3 leaves like the ones shown here, stay away!

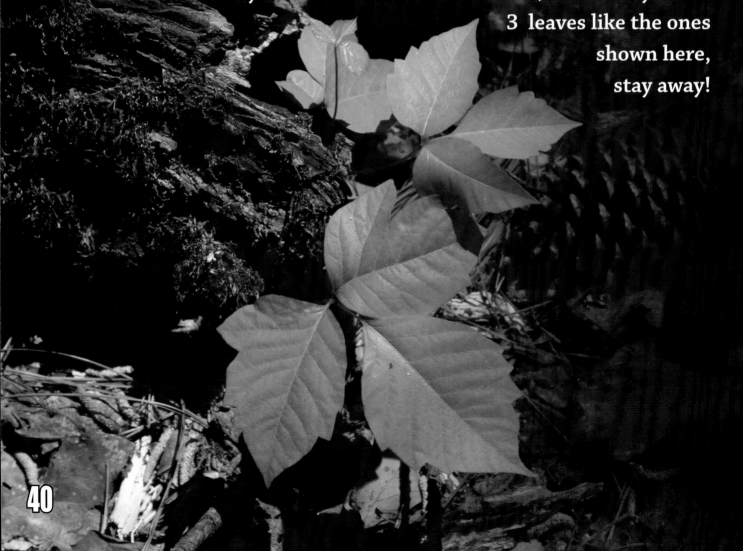

Insects are also a source of allergens for some people. One of the most common indoor allergies is triggered by cockroaches. Doctors believe cockroaches are responsible for most cases of asthma in children who live in cities. The allergen comes from the cockroaches' feces (poop) and saliva.

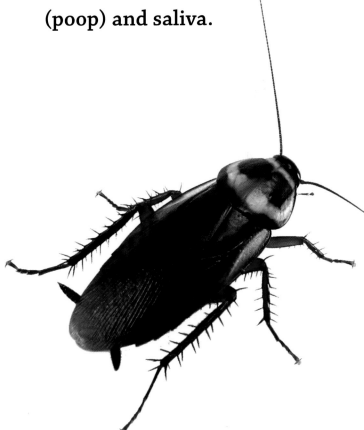

If you're not allergic to bee stings, and you get stung, you'll probably have a sore bump from the sting—but people with an allergy to bee stings have extreme reactions. Their throats can swell shut, getting in the way of their breathing. People with this allergy often have to carry emergency treatment with them. This can save their lives.

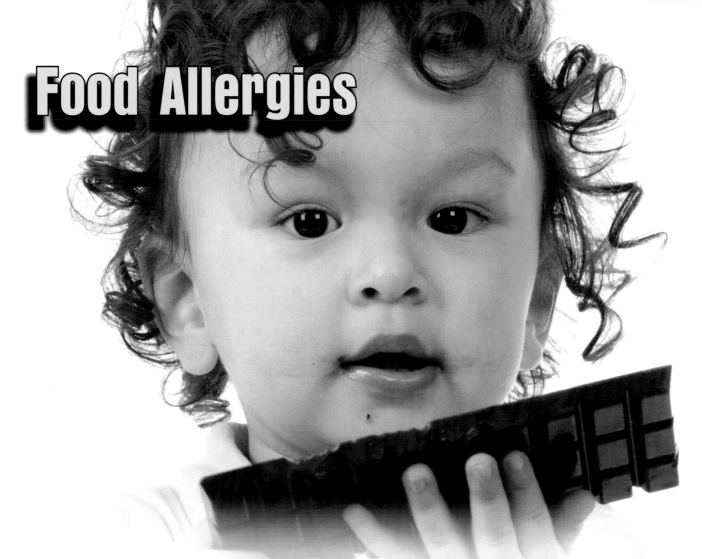

Food Allergies

Food allergies are triggered by certain foods. Symptoms can include: a tingling feeling in the mouth, swelling of the tongue and the throat, difficulty breathing, hives, vomiting, stomach cramps, and diarrhea. These symptoms usually appear within minutes to two hours after the person has eaten the food.

Many different kinds of food can trigger allergies, but the most common are:

- milk
- eggs
- peanuts
- tree nuts
- fish
- shellfish
- soy
- wheat

Food allergies can trigger anaphylaxis, a serious allergic reaction that happens quickly and may cause death.

If you have a food allergy, it's important to avoid the foods to which you're allergic. Food allergies can be very serious, even life-threatening.

Words to Know

Life-threatening: capable of causing death.

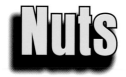 Nuts

Peanut allergies can be mild—or severe. People with serious peanut allergies can react to even tiny pieces of peanut, such as those found in packaged foods that were manufactured in factories that also make foods containing peanuts. Even though peanuts may not be on these foods' ingredients list, those infinitesimal specks of peanut are enough to make some people very sick.

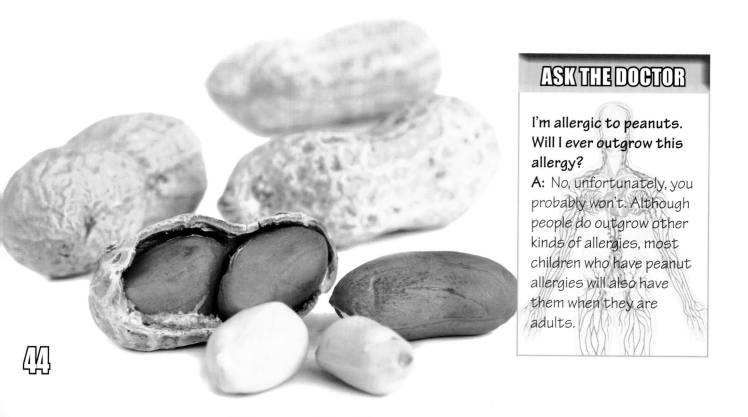

ASK THE DOCTOR

I'm allergic to peanuts. Will I ever outgrow this allergy?

A: No, unfortunately, you probably won't. Although people do outgrow other kinds of allergies, most children who have peanut allergies will also have them when they are adults.

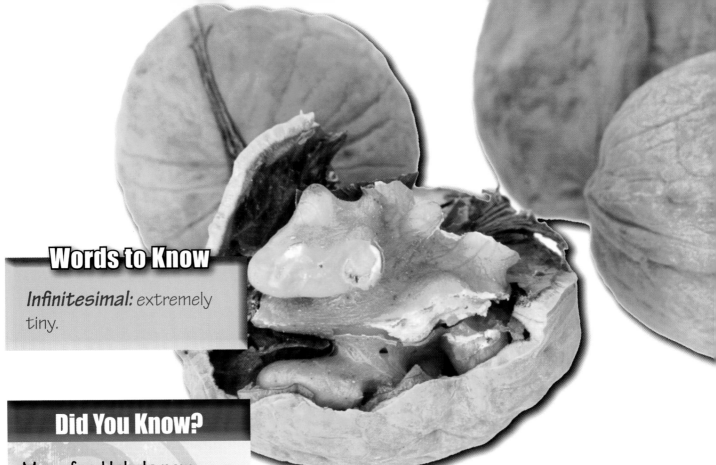

Did You Know?

Many food labels now carry these warnings:

• "may contain nuts"

• "produced on shared equipment with nuts or peanuts"

• "produced in a facility that also processes nuts"

If you're allergic to peanuts, there's greater chance that you'll be allergic to tree nuts (like the walnuts shown here) as well. If you have a nut allergy, you need to be careful to read ingredients. Many cookies, cakes, and ice cream contain nuts.

Eggs

Most people who are allergic to eggs react to the proteins in egg whites, but some people are also allergic to the proteins in the yolk. Egg allergy usually first appears when kids are very young. The good news is that most kids outgrow it by the time they're 5 years old.

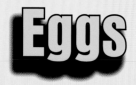

Words to Know

Respiratory: having to do with breathing.

Did You Know?

For people who are especially sensitive to eggs, even egg fumes or getting egg on the skin can cause a serious anaphylactic reaction. If someone in a household has a serious allergy like this, eggs should be kept out of the house completely.

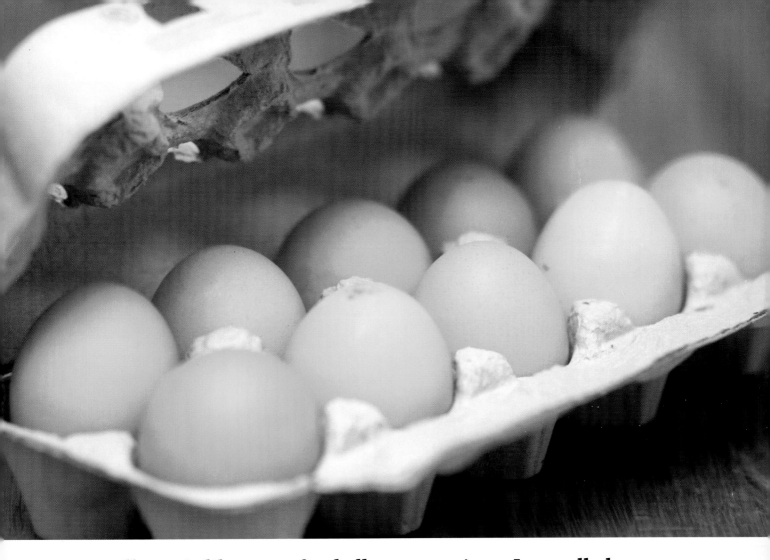

Egg allergy is like most food allergy reactions: It usually happens within minutes to hours after eating eggs. Most reactions last less than a day and may affect any of three body systems: the skin, the digestive system, or the respiratory system.

Milk

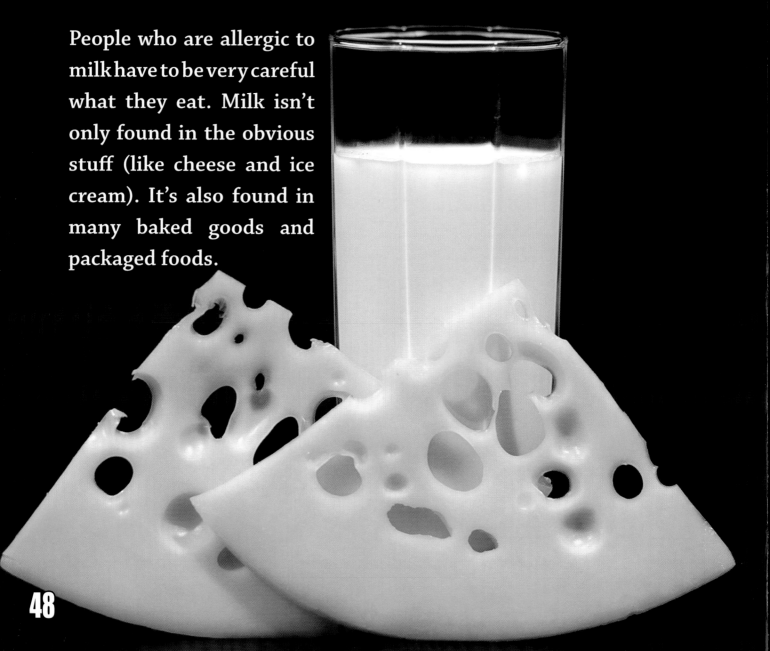

People who are allergic to milk have to be very careful what they eat. Milk isn't only found in the obvious stuff (like cheese and ice cream). It's also found in many baked goods and packaged foods.

People often confuse milk allergies with another condition called "lactose intolerance," but they're not at all the same thing. Lactose intolerance involves the digestive system, not the immune system. A person with lactose intolerance can't digest the sugars in milk, but a person with a milk allergy has an immune reaction to the proteins found in milk.

Words to Know

Intolerance: lacking an ability to stand something.

Did You Know?

Milk products contain calcium and vitamin D, both of which your body needs for good health. If you're allergic to milk, you need to be careful to get these nutrients from other foods. In some countries, orange juice and other juices are fortified now with calcium to help kids with milk allergies.

Fish

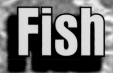

Some allergies start during childhood (and some go away in adulthood). Fish allergies, however, are most apt to start when a person is grown up. People who are allergic to fish will have an itchy reaction in their mouth and throat if they eat fish. They are also more apt to have asthma.

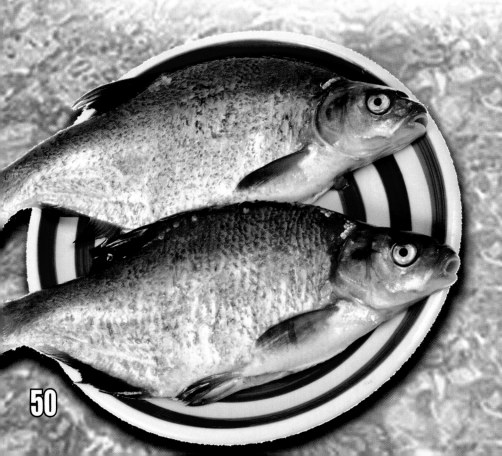

Did You Know?

These foods may contain fish:

- Worcestershire sauce
- Caesar salad
- caviar
- Imitation seafood (often used in sushi)

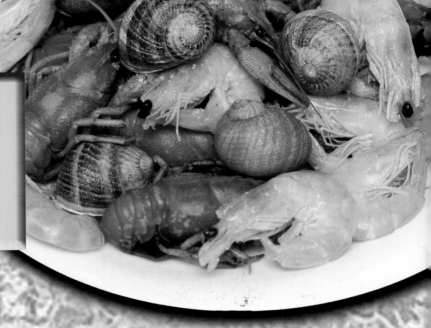

Many people who are allergic to fish are also allergic to shellfish. It's fairly easy to avoid these foods, but as with nuts, sometimes something called "cross-contamination" happens during food preparation. This could happen at a restaurant, for instance, where a hamburger or french fries were fried in the same oil used to fry fish. Tiny allergens from the fish might end up on the meat or french fries, triggering a reaction in the person who sits down to eat thinking he's avoided eating anything that resembles a fish.

Fruit

Unlike other food allergies, fruit allergies are seldom very serious. Many people, however, get an itchy, burning feeling in their mouths when they eat certain fruits.

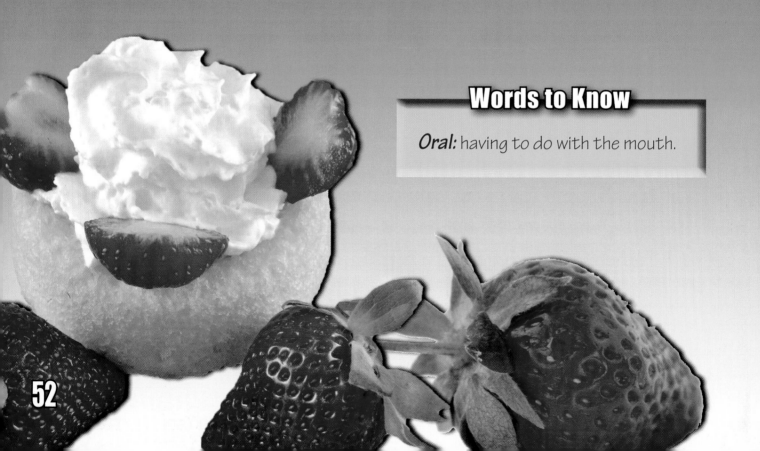

Words to Know

Oral: having to do with the mouth.

Scientists have discovered that people who have this reaction to fruits are also allergic to certain kinds of pollen. It's called "cross-reactivity." The chemicals in some fruits are so similar to the chemicals in some pollen that a person with an allergy responds in the same way to both things. If you're allergic to pollen from birch trees, for example, you're more apt to have an oral allergy to apples, pears, peaches, plums, apricots, cherries, hazelnuts, and kiwis. People with ragweed allergies are more prone to have an oral reaction to the gourd family (watermelon, squash, cucumber). Peeling or slightly heating the fruit may be all you need to do to be able to eat fruit again.

Did You Know?

Citrus fruit (like oranges, lemons, and grapefruit) and berries do not cause oral allergies.

How Do You Know If You Have An Allergy?

If you think you might have an allergy, talk to a doctor. (A doctor who deals only with allergies is called an allergist.) The doctor may ask you questions like these: What are your symptoms? How long have they been going on? Do other people in your family have allergies? What makes the symptoms better? What makes them worse? Are you taking any medication now?

If you think you might have a food allergy, the allergist may suggest an elimination diet. Foods that might trigger allergies are cut out from your diet for a period of time, perhaps a few weeks. Then, one at a time, those foods will be put back into your diet. You will need to pay close attention to any symptoms you experience during this time. Anything that may have triggered a reaction will then be withdrawn again, to see if the symptoms clear up.

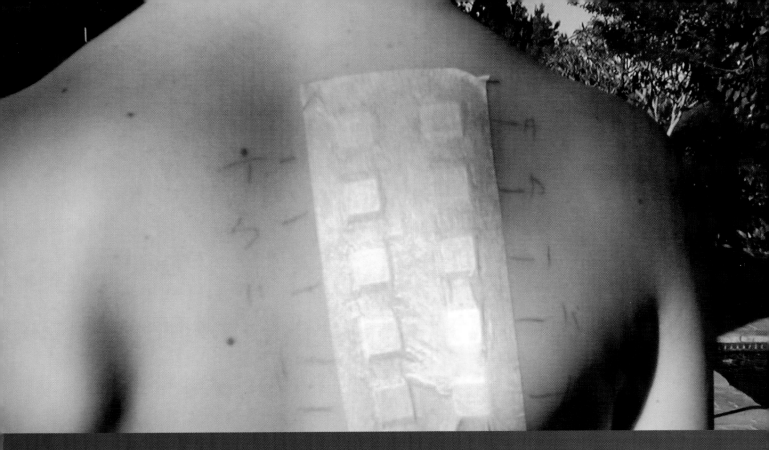

Words to Know

Symptoms: the physical signs that a disease or other condition is going on.

Elimination: the act of getting rid of something.

Diagnosed: decided what disease or condition is causing a set of symptoms.

Allergies can be diagnosed with a skin test like the one shown above. Each square of skin has been scratched with a different possible allergen. If any squares show a reaction (become red or swollen), it means an allergy is present to that substance.

What Should You Do If You Have An Allergy?

If your doctor decides you have an allergy, she may want you to take medicine. Medications called antihistamines counteract allergic reactions. Some of these medicines are available over-the-counter at a drugstore, while others need a prescription from your doctor.

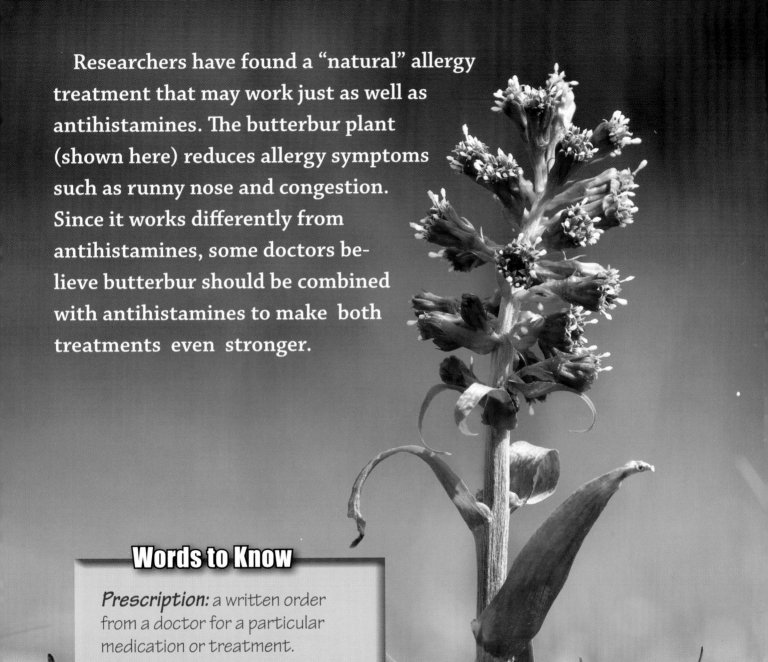

Researchers have found a "natural" allergy treatment that may work just as well as antihistamines. The butterbur plant (shown here) reduces allergy symptoms such as runny nose and congestion. Since it works differently from antihistamines, some doctors believe butterbur should be combined with antihistamines to make both treatments even stronger.

Words to Know

Prescription: a written order from a doctor for a particular medication or treatment.

57

Real Kids

Can one person make a difference? Kelsey Ryan did. Kelsey is a 9-year-old who is allergic to peanuts. If she eats a peanut or anything with peanut oil on it, she can die from anaphylactic shock. The only thing that stops the allergic reaction is the drug epinephrine, so Kelsey carries an EpiPen® with her wherever she goes. (The EpiPen® is a needle-like device that allows her to give herself a quick shot of epinephrine.)

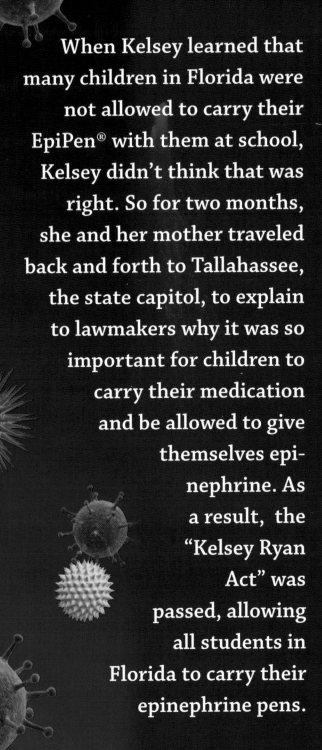

When Kelsey learned that many children in Florida were not allowed to carry their EpiPen® with them at school, Kelsey didn't think that was right. So for two months, she and her mother traveled back and forth to Tallahassee, the state capitol, to explain to lawmakers why it was so important for children to carry their medication and be allowed to give themselves epi-nephrine. As a result, the "Kelsey Ryan Act" was passed, allowing all students in Florida to carry their epinephrine pens.

Find Out More

These Web sites will tell you more about allergies:

Allergies
allergies.com

Allergies: Things You Can Do to Control Your Symptoms
familydoctor.org/083.xml

eMedicine: Food Allergies
www.emedicine.com/med/TOPIC806.HT

Kids' Health: Allergies
www.kidshealth.org/teen/diseases_conditions/ allergies_immune/
allergies.html

Mayo Clinic Allergy Center
www.mayoclinic.com/health/allergy/AA99999

MedlinePlus: Allergies
www.nlm.nih.gov/medlineplus/allergy.htm

World Allergy Organization
www.worldallergy.org/links.php

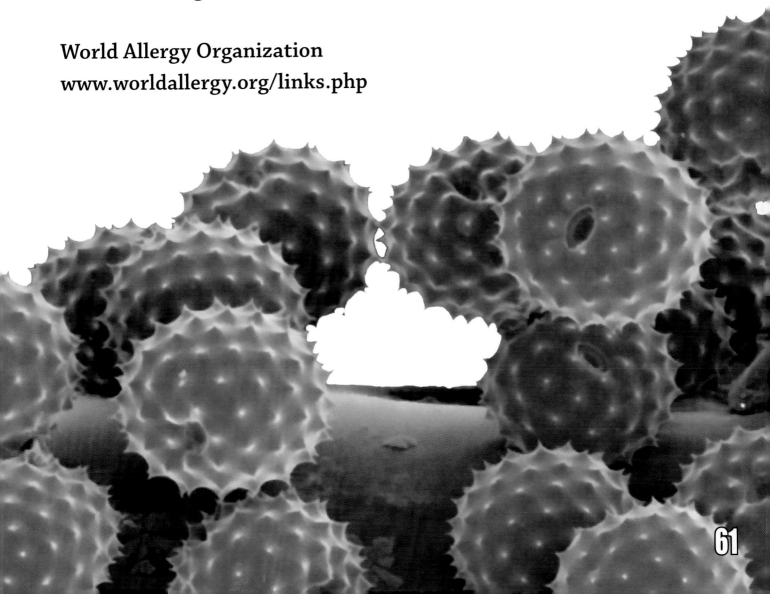

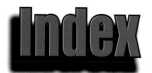

Index

Picture Credits

American Academy of Allergy, Asthma, & Immunology: p. 19
Archives of Pediatric and Adolescent Medicine: p. 19
Asthma & Respiratory Foundation: p. 47

Dreamstime
Artproem: p. 45
Baronskie: p. 33
Bobelia: p. 30
Darren: p. 10
Eraxion: pp. 12, 18
Henrischmit: pp. 24–25
ImagePoint Photos: p. 16
Jirsta: p. 17
KrishnaCreations: p. 15
Millann: p. 39
Moori: p. 43

Pelvidge: p. 32
Prawny: p. 59
Rbouwman: p. 34
Rolffimages: pp. 26–27
Stuart Key: p. 46
Stuart Miles: p. 20
Whitechild: pp. 8–9, 57
Stuart Key: p. 46
Stuart Miles: p. 20
Whitechild: pp. 8–9, 57
EMS: p. 46
EPA: p. 13
Georgia Tech/Gary Meck: p. 48
Jupiter Images: pp. 22–23, 28, 36, 37, 52, 54, 55
New Scientist: p. 21
New York City Dept. of Health & Mental Hygiene Asthma Campaign: p. 41
Wikipedia: p. 29
World Asthma Foundation: pp. 50–51

To the best knowledge of the publisher, all other images are in the public domain. If any image has been inadvertently uncredited, please notify Harding House Publishing Service, Vestal, New York 13850, so that rectification can be made for future printings.

About the Author

Rae Simons has written many books for young adults and children. She lives with her family in New York State in the U.S.

About the Consultant

Elise DeVore Berlan, MD, MPH, FAAP, is a faculty member of the Division of Adolescent Health at Nationwide Children's Hospital and an Assistant Professor of Clinical Pediatrics at The Ohio State University College of Medicine. She completed her Fellowship in Adolescent Medicine at Children's Hospital Boston and obtained a Master's Degree in Public Health at the Harvard School of Public Health. Dr. Berlan completed her residency in pediatrics at the Children's Hospital of Philadelphia, where she also served an additional year as Chief Resident. She received her medical degree from the University of Iowa College of Medicine.